GUNPOWDER AS A WAR REMEDY

A WORK OF HOMEOPATHY

First Edition 1915
John H Clarke MD

New Edition 2016
Edited by Tarl Warwick

COPYRIGHT AND DISCLAIMER

The first edition of this work is in the public domain having been written prior to 1923. This edition, with its cover art and format, is all rights reserved.

In no way may this text be construed as encouraging or condoning any harmful or illegal act. In no way may this text be construed as able to diagnose, treat, cure, or prevent any disease, injury, symptom, or condition.

GUNPOWDER AS A WAR REMEDY

FOREWORD

The following work was crafted at the dawn of the 20th century by John H Clarke; an interesting and eclectic man, once the leader of a nationalistic movement and a fervent homeopath and competent author of some dozens of works, some rather significant, such as his *Materia Medica* (spoken of within this selfsame text.) Unfortunately, Clarke has been tarred with the same brush as so many others within his era as an "antisemite" for espousing views so common at the time that they were scarcely challenged at all anywhere in the world. That he died in 1931 and was a man of the first, not second, world war, seems to be a statement lacking in most literature about him.

"Gunpowder" however is not a social manifesto but an interesting medical text which might actually have some significance; Clarke correctly identifies the antiseptic capabilities of saltpeter and sulfur, and proposes that standard black powder (as opposed to manufactured smokeless powder now almost solely used outside of the stone mining or historical arms industries) is a cure specifically for infections, boils, blood poisoning, and other maladies. For the former this is probably correct outside of life threatening infections; applied topically or perhaps, as he states, taken in ingested form. As for its usefulness in treating the after-effects of inhaling sewer gas (possibly hydrogen sulfide or carbon monoxide) or syphilis, I suppose a bit more skepticism is called for regardless of his claims.

We see here an interesting treatment of what, specifically, was considered as well to cause illness to begin with; "germ theory" here is spoken of as an actual theory rather than an established and observable fact (in the early 20th century this is not odd) and earthquake dust is apparently considered to cause skin ailments.

GUNPOWDER AS A WAR REMEDY

Clarke's specific remedy is a tincture taken from gunpowder itself in a more standardized form and with a lower overall concentration- apparently from 1/10 concentration to 1/1,000 concentration; it is not clear that such a small amount of gunpowder dissolved and purified into solution would be capable of significant chemical action, even if we regard the constituents of the same to be medically active. Sulfur destroys some bacteria, Saltpeter certainly does the same. Black carbon has a variety of medical uses and is often crushed into a sort of drink and given to those with alcohol poisoning to flush their system of remaining alcohol. I have found personally that claims of it whitening teeth are nonsense, but it does remove coffee or tobacco stains from the same and thus the user will see some restoration of normal color.

It should be noted that this text was produced during the Great War- world war one. Therefore, when Clarke indicates that he has sent some of his remedy off to the "front" he literally means to the trenches. It is not clear whether his homeopathy was able to save those there in the trenches from foot rot and trench fever or other maladies, but the general lack of medical knowledge in this period renders his solutions at least as helpful as what was generally doled out to soldiers at the time.

This edition of "Gunpowder as a War Remedy" has been edited into fully modern English usage and several errors in grammar have been corrected. Care has been taken to retain the original intent and meaning of all passages.

GUNPOWDER AS A WAR REMEDY

PREFACE

My authority having been cited in the Evening Standard, Daily Mirror, and other journals for the recommendation of Gunpowder as an all-around remedy for blood poisoning in general and septic war wounds in particular, I think I shall best serve the public interest by putting the facts about the remedy into separate practical shape and thus making them accessible to all.

In the following pamphlet will be found all the information necessary for the practical use and understanding of the remedy, and I think that the directions are so clear and simple that any intelligent person, lay or medical, will be able to put them into practice.

John H Clarke.

CONTENTS

CH. 1 – How Gunpowder is to be taken.

CH. 2 – The constitution and therapeutic power of gunpowder.

CH. 3 – Examples of the curative action of gunpowder.

CH. 4 – Concluding remarks.

GUNPOWDER AS A WAR REMEDY

CHAPTER I

So much interest has been evoked by an article of mine which appeared in the Homoeopathic World of January last, entitled "Gunpowder for Gunners," that I have thought well to write out a full account of Gunpowder in this somewhat novel aspect of its many utilities, which, so far as history tells, was undreamed of by its discoverer, the alchemist friar, Roger Bacon.

The Form In Which It May Be Taken

In the first place it may be advisable to say a few words about the form in which the remedy may be taken. In the old days of black powder, gunpowder was recognized by our soldiers as a remedy for certain forms of suppuration, and by them it was taken crude in teaspoonful doses mixed in hot water.

It is also used crude by shepherds, as the Rector of Stradbroke has told us, sprinkled on bread and cheese, to cure and prevent wound-poisoning acquired in shearing and handling sheep. But crude gunpowder is neither a convenient nor a pleasant remedy to take, though I have no authority for stating that it would not be efficacious.

The preparation I have most frequently used is the homoeopathic third decimal (3x) trituration, either prescribed in the form of powders or of compressed tablets. For war purposes the last are the most convenient. In this form I find gunpowder a most powerful and efficacious remedy.

The 3x trituration is what is called a "low attenuation",

GUNPOWDER AS A WAR REMEDY

that is to say, it is not highly infinitesimal but it is sufficiently so to have lost all taste or smell of crude gunpowder, and to be in no sort of way explosive.

Dosage And Directions For Use

The great sphere of action of gunpowder is in cases of septic suppuration or, in other words of wounds that have become poisoned with the germs of putrefaction.

My directions in such cases areas follows:

One tablet every two hours when there is fever.

Two tablets three or four times a day when the temperature is normal.

But Gunpowder may also be used as a prophylactic.

That is to say, it will not only cure septic suppuration when present, but it will afford such protection to the organism against harmful germs, that wounds will be less likely to become septic in one who is under its influence. For this purpose I recommend:

As a prophylactic one tablet to be taken once a day.

Judging from analogy I should expect that this would also afford protection against other forms of blood-poisoning as well as against poisoned wounds. One tablet of Gunpowder a day is no hardship or difficulty for anybody. I should think it ought to prove effective against the infection of spotted fever, or cerebro-spinal meningitis.

If this disease actually appears in any locality, I should advise all who are quartered in that locality to take:

One tablet three times a day.

In the case of boils, carbuncles, and other skin affections, including eczema, abscesses, whether septic or non blood poisoning from bites of insects, ptomaine poisoning from food that has been improperly preserved, I should prescribe:

One tablet every hour or two hours according to the urgency of the symptoms.

The same dosage would apply in the case of illness from any of the protective inoculations or vaccinations that are now in such vogue. The portability of the remedy in this form is another recommendation in its favor. An ounce bottle contains 160 tablets.

Thus, without perceptibly adding to the weight or bulk of his kit any soldier can carry with him as much as he is likely to need. Any homoeopathic chemist will be able to supply the tablets. My own chemists, Messrs. Epps, 60 Jermyn Street, S.W., have already sent out a quantity to the front.

CHAPTER II

The Gunpowder with which we are concerned is the traditional Black Gunpowder, whose three cardinal constituents are sulfur, carbon, and niter or saltpeter. Modern smokeless

GUNPOWDER AS A WAR REMEDY

gunpowder is of a different composition.

As sulfur, carbon, and saltpeter are three potent medicines well known to pharmacy and physic, it is not surprising that a combination of the three should also be a medicine of great potency. There is a certain piquancy in the fact that gunpowder is a remedy for the accidents of warfare; but some instinct put into the minds of our soldiers of long ago that gunpowder could cure as well as kill.

The Indians of North America and Canada have found in it a remedy for snake-bites. The shepherds of East Anglia, as already mentioned, use it extensively in treating their flocks and themselves for wounds and blood-poisoning of many kinds, and for protecting themselves against wound infection.

In the second volume of my Dictionary of *Materia Medica*, published in 1902, I have referred to some uses of Gunpowder in my article on Saltpeter ("Kalium nitricum"), recording also some experiments made with it on myself. But my knowledge of the power of Gunpowder over blood poisoning I owe to a graphic article contributed to the Homoeopathic World in 1911 by the Rector of Stradbroke, Suffolk, the Rev. Roland Upcher, entitled "Notes on the Use of Gunpowder (Black)."

"For the last forty years," wrote Mr. Upcher, "I have known and observed from personal experiment the effects of Black Gunpowder as a remedy for various kinds of blood poisoning. The symptoms of poisoning which call for Black Gunpowder are almost invariably abscesses or boils or carbuncles, and frequently, though not always, exaggerated swelling of the poisoned limb, accompanied with discoloration

GUNPOWDER AS A WAR REMEDY

of the skin, so that the arm from the tips of the fingers to the axillary glands is almost of a purple or black tint. In such cases I have found Black Gunpowder, whether in large or small doses, acts like magic."

Mr. Upcher tells the story of how he came by the discovery:

"My father, a country rector in Norfolk, used to add to his light duties in a small parish the recreation of farming the glebe, and as there was a good lot of pasture, kept sheep. He noticed that at the time of paring the sheeps' feet suffering from foot-rot, his shepherds were continually subjected to blood poisoning, which was more or less (less, I fear!) successfully treated by local doctors. But it generally ended in the said shepherd having to give up his work and turn his hand to something else. However, at last there came a shepherd, who, year in and year out, never did get blood-poisoning!"

This greatly astonished the rector, and he asked his shepherd how be accounted for the fact. The latter invited his master to come and see him at his afternoon meal, or "fourses" as the Norfolk people call it. He duly went, and found him sitting under a hedge eating bread and what looked like black cheese.

"Why, Harry," he exclaimed, "whatever are you eating? It looks like black cheese."

"No, master," was the reply, " that b'aint black cheese, but that is white cheese kivered with black gunpowder, and that's what keeps out the pison, that's what dew the trick- I never gets no pison."

GUNPOWDER AS A WAR REMEDY

In course of time this shepherd got promoted to a better position, and his successor soon got into trouble when the feet-paring season came round. The shepherd's arm was swollen and almost black from finger-tips to armpit. The Rector did not trouble the faculty this time, but undertook the case himself.

He mixed a dessertspoonful of gunpowder in half a tumbler of water, making a paste of it first, and gradually adding he water afterwards, and administered the whole in one dose!

Result: A brilliant and rapid cure.

From that time on the Rector's shepherds took gunpowder with their cheese, and blood-poisoning disappeared. But the lesson did not stop there. The Rector could not keep a good thing like that to himself, and as in duty bound, let his parish have the benefit of the discovery.

"Many a time," says his son, "have I been dosed, as a child, boy, and even young man, with the family patent medicine: boils, carbuncles, eruptions caused by suspected blood poisoning, one and all had to climb down to the Black Gunpowder."

As with the family so with the parish-all conditions of men, women, and children, and even animals, were treated by the good Rector with the same remedy and the same success. Rector ll., the present Mr. Upcher, used the homoeopathic preparation of Gunpowder- the one with which I experimented on myself. This is at once more convenient and more pleasant than crude Gunpowder, and no less potent for curative purposes. From my knowledge of the properties of sulfur, carbon, and

GUNPOWDER AS A WAR REMEDY

saltpeter individually, I had no doubt whatever that the observations of the shepherds and their spiritual pastors were thoroughly sound.

The whole art of curative medicine may be said to lie in one thing- correctly reading indications.

When a case presents itself for treatment, there are generally a hundred remedies more or less applicable to the case. In order to select the best of the bunch, it is essential to be able to read correctly the manifestations signs and symptoms of the patient.

It is very easy to make too much of one symptom and too little of another, and so miss the particular drug that is required. Now the great point about Gunpowder is that it has a broad and clear indication that hardly anyone can miss- blood poisoning.

Soldiers found it; shepherds found it; American Indians found it. An ordinary cut or wound in a healthy person heals quickly, but if a morbid virus is introduced, or if the person's blood is impure or of low vitality, the part swells, suppuration ensues, and the limb may be threatened.

Or if a limb is bitten by a poisonous snake, the same thing happens, only more rapidly, and the constitutional symptoms are more rapid, in development. Or, poisonous matter of some kind may be introduced into the system by other ways- breathing foul air, drinking polluted water, or eating tainted food. The poison quickly finds its way into the blood-boils, carbuncles, eruptions, abscesses, or other manifestations appear,

GUNPOWDER AS A WAR REMEDY

showing unmistakably that the blood has been poisoned.

To all these conditions Gunpowder acts as an antidote. It may be asked, In what way does it act? Does it exercise an antiseptic action and kill the germs? In a certain degree there is some such action.

Carbon and sulfur, with sulfur derivatives such as sulfurous acid, are very potent antiseptics and germ destroyers. But the amount of these taken in the preparations used in my cases is quite insufficient to exert a direct germ-killing action. But Gunpowder, in the homoeopathic attenuation, so acts on the blood as to render it antiseptic, or, more strictly speaking, to assist or increase its normal antiseptic action. For the healthy living blood is a potent germ destroyer, and the reason why all persons do not succumb to infection when epidemics are abroad is that the blood of those who escape is equal to killing the germs which attack them.

It may be asked: How can an infinitesimal amount of Gunpowder, or of anything else for that matter, effect this? To answer this fully one would need to explain the secret of life itself. However, we know a good deal about life; and the phenomena connected with Radium are capable of throwing a little light on the subject.

Substances, when undergoing the process of graduated attenuation of the homoeopathic method, while losing their coarse physical properties, acquire others which are somewhat closely analogous to the properties of radium. In this way; a substance which has been in contact with radium, through the action of the radium rays, becomes itself radiant.

GUNPOWDER AS A WAR REMEDY

So, the homoeopathically attenuated substances are raised to a higher pitch of vibration and become capable of conveying their vibrations to the persons who take them, just as radium can convey its vibrations to bodies in contact with it. Be this as it may (and it must be confessed that all attempted "explanations" of the phenomena of life are at bottom unsatisfying), the fact remains that Gunpowder, taken in minute quantities, enables the blood to get rid of disease germs which the constituents of Gunpowder in substantial amounts would kill if added to the same in a test-tube. Fortunately, it is facts and not explanations that we have to deal with.

Most explanations amount to little more than a re-statement of the problem in different terms, which are constantly changing. But the facts remain the same always for our use and constant guidance. It may be asked, What about antiseptics? Are not they sufficient?

Now, I have no sort of objection to antiseptics in themselves. Antiseptic, or, rather, aseptic surgery, is a very great advance on older methods, but the use of antiseptics is largely dependent on the germ-theory, and the germ-theory is only one side of the question. The vital question is the other and, as I think, the larger side.

The cases in which it is impossible to keep or make wounds aseptic by external applications are innumerable. Besides, it is quite possible to hinder healing by their use. For in order to kill any germs present in a wound it may be necessary to apply an antiseptic in such strength as to lower the vitality of the injured part.

GUNPOWDER AS A WAR REMEDY

This explains why many wounds refuse to heal under the most careful antiseptic treatment, it is for this reason that the practice of so acting on the blood as to increase its own vitality is infinitely superior. For local dressings I prefer plain sterilized lint after cleansing with pure boiled water, or better still, with pure boiled water in which tincture of Calendula (the Common Marigold) or of Hamamelis (Witch Hazel) has been mixed in the proportion of a teaspoonful to the half-pint. These are very useful adjuncts; but the internal remedy is the main thing, and this will act in spite of all sorts of unfavorable conditions.

Mr. Roland Upcher began his experiments with Gunpowder itself, and then followed these with the lower homoeopathic preparations:

The 1X trituration is equal to 0.1 in the decimal scale; 2X is 0.01, and 3X is 0.001, or one thousandth part of the crude. Mr. Upcher gives his reasons for believing in the therapeutic virtues of Gunpowder by a consideration of the individual properties of its constituents.

After remarking that sulfur is a well-known remedy for boils, eruptions, itch, eczema, and suppressed impurities and eruptions; that carbon (Carbo vegetabilis) covers very similar ground; that saltpeter (Kali nitricum) has a powerful action on the skin, opening the pores; he quotes the following passage from my Dictionary of *Materia Medica*, Vol. II., page 144:

"A solution of saltpeter as an application was an old remedy for inveterate mange in cats. Saltpeter with carbon and sulfur forms Gunpowder. A teaspoonful of this in hot water was a favorite remedy for gonorrhea among soldiers in the days when black gunpowder was used. In some experiments made by myself with Gunpowder 2X severe herpes facialis involving right eyebrow and right side of the nose developed."

Mr. Upcher adds that from his experience of Gunpowder in the cure of herpes, he can verify the correctness of my experiment on myself. In selecting Gunpowder 3X for my therapeutic work instead of lower attenuation I have perhaps been influenced by the experiment above alluded to.

I carry the marks of it to the present day, and I have no wish to repeat the experiment on anyone else. Gunpowder 3X has hitherto answered my expectations without causing any unpleasant by-results.

CHAPTER III

In addition to the cases related by Mr. Upcher it may be of interest to record a few of my own. First, I will give that of the gunner, whose case I related in the article already referred to. It will be noticed that in this case I gave other remedies besides Gunpowder, but the progress of the case showed that the Gunpowder was the chief agent in the curative work.

H.J.S., 30, a non-commissioned artillery officer in an Indian regiment, who had been born in India of English parents, and had never before left it, presented himself to me on April 9th, 1913, in a fairly desperate condition.

He was a man of very powerful physique, but his flesh was hanging about him, and he was covered from head to foot with sores, some discharging, some having rupia-like crusts,

GUNPOWDER AS A WAR REMEDY

copper colored stains marking the areas where sores or "boils" had previously been.

His story was as follows. About two years before he had had an outbreak of "boils," and six months later another attack. At intervals of four or five months he had other attacks, ending up with the present one. All attempts to cure him having failed, he was advised that the only thing for him was a voyage to England and a change of air. H.J.S. was greatly valued by his superiors. He was an instructor in athletics, a total abstainer, and an expert gunner.

In order that he might not lose his pay whilst absent from India, his officers had very kindly arranged for him a course of instruction at Woolwich. He had been six weeks in England when he came to me. So far from the change benefiting him, he had become steadily worse. He had had diarrhea during the voyage home.

His digestion was bad and his sleep broken by the pains of his sores. He had lost two stones in weight in four weeks; altogether he had lost five stones.

The neck, trunk, extremities were all affected.

The inguinal glands were much swollen and painful. On trying to get at the origin of the trouble, I ascertained that his previous health had been excellent. But in 1894 he had been bitten in the finger by a squirrel and his finger had been bad for a long time afterwards. This showed a degree of susceptibility to blood-poisoning. He had had attacks of fever, but almost always in association with the attacks of "boils."

GUNPOWDER AS A WAR REMEDY

The first attack occurred the end of November, 1911.

At the end of the previous October he had been vaccinated, for the second time in his life, and it "took well."

It did, indeed! To me, the connection was obvious between the present state and the vaccination. At the same time as my patient, a fellow soldier was also vaccinated, and he also soon afterwards became ill, in a somewhat similar way. But this man was not temperate in his habits, and his illness was put down to alcohol by his medical officers.

This would not do for my patient, who was a life abstainer. The only other hypothesis was syphilis. The possibility of this he steadily denied, and his word was borne out by the Wassermann tests, which consistently gave negative results, though tried again and again.

My diagnosis was unhesitatingly- Vaccinosis- secondary or tertiary. This was confirmed by the fact that the sores were thickest and lasted longest on his right arm on the site of the vaccination scars. The fact that his right arm was worse, was explained by his doctors as being due to over-exertion at cricket, bowling, etc!

I ordered him Gunpowder 3X eight grains three times a day; and Thuja 200 three doses in the week. At the end of the week he was a changed man. He had still plenty of sores, but they were healing, and the whole aspect of the man was different, his appetite had improved to such an extent that some indigestion and diarrhea had resulted from overindulgence. His skin had improved altogether in appearance.

GUNPOWDER AS A WAR REMEDY

On April 24th his weight was 10st 11lbs. He had then gained much, but I have no record of his weight when he first came to me. On June 5th he was 11st. 11 1/2 lbs. and on September 18th, 12st. 6 1/2 lbs.

He had steadily improved all this time. New swellings or "boils" occasionally appeared, and some sores with thickening on the hands, just below the wrists, especially the right, had proved particularly obstinate. I now omitted Gunpowder and gave instead Silica 3X in eight-grain doses in the same way; Thuja 200, thrice a week, being continued as before.

A rapid change took place. A new outbreak of boils occurred, diarrhea set in, with bitter taste and coated tongue and some fever. The diarrhea was worse after drinking milk.

The weight had gone down to 11st 8lbs., but the hands were much better. Trombid. 200 soon cured the diarrhea, and then I gave Gunpowder 3X eight grains every four hours alone; leaving off the Thuja. On October 16th he was very much better again in every way, his weight having gone up to 12st. 2 1/2 lbs. Soon after this, his time being expired, he left for India after successfully completing his course of instruction, in very good condition.

I gave him a good supply of Gunpowder to take home with him, and told him to let me know if he had any relapse. As I have heard nothing since, I conclude he is now busy with his guns somewhere in the widespread area of the war.

Here are a few other cases of mine:

GUNPOWDER AS A WAR REMEDY

Poisoned Bite

A lady, who had a very sensitive skin, was bitten by a gnat on the foot, resulting in swelling, inflammation and suppuration. There was a ring of inflammation round the bite, constantly spreading and detaching the epidermis as it spread. After the failure of several remedies, Gunpowder 3X eight grains three times a day rapidly cured.

Poisoned Cut

A gentleman had a bad cut with a knife on the left index finger. The wound refused to heal.

An inflammatory ring stripped off the epidermis and spread more and more. Lachesis and other remedies failed to make any impression. Gunpowder 3X rapidly cured.

Sewer-Gas Poisoning

A lady was very severely poisoned by sewer gas. There followed swelling of the right arm and axillary glands of the right side.

When she consulted me, three months after the accident, the right arm was almost fixed at the elbow-joint with swelling. It threatened suppuration above and below. The axillary glands were as large as a hen's egg.

Gunpowder 3X gradually resolved the trouble, and though the cure was interrupted by an attack of measles, the mobility of the arm was fully restored.

GUNPOWDER AS A WAR REMEDY

The following case shows that as earthquakes and war are placed in the same category of calamities, Gunpowder may prove of service in some of the ills caused by the one as well as the other.

Blood-Poisoning From Earthquake Dust

In 1912 I had under my care a lady who had been in the great earthquake which wrought so much havoc in Jamaica some years before. She asked me if I thought I could do anything for her little niece, aged 4, who lived in Jamaica and suffered from a skin trouble. She was born soon after the earthquake, was a very tiny child, had always been nervous, and suffered, as many other children of the colony have done since the earthquake, from eruptions on the skin.

It was as if the earthquake had thrown up from the depths some new kind of irritant and poisonous dust.

The first symptoms were "prickly heat," with much itching. Then sores appeared, forming blisters, the fluid of which had to be let out.

The parts affected were chiefly the ankles and the trunk. Every mosquito bite made a poisoned wound. This little patient was very languid, was nervous at night, and a restless sleeper. These were the facts I elicited from her aunt.

I thought Gunpowder was the very thing for her, and on January 4th, 1912, I sent her a supply of powders of the 5X. In due course I received a report that within a week or commencing the remedy she was much better. She slept better, the bowels acted better, and as for her appetite, whereas formerly she had to be coaxed to eat anything, now they could not give her enough. The skin improved at the same time.

A second course of powders was sent on April 30th as there had been a relapse of the eruption with fever. From this time she steadily improved and got perfectly well. I may append to these an Editorial note from the Homoeopathic World of June 1st, relating the work of another observer:

Septic Inflammation Of Thumb

"More Gunpowder cases continue to come to hand. The latest is of a septic inflammation of the thumb in a nurse of 19. It was vigorously treated surgically, and pus evacuated, but the inflammation continued, and the loss of a joint was contemplated until a short course of Gunpowder 3X achieved a satisfactory healing and scarring."

CHAPTER IV

I think it will be agreed that the evidence adduced above is sufficient to warrant my recommendation of Gunpowder as a remedy of almost universal applicability in wounds of war. It has the additional advantage of being, in the form recommended, whilst powerful for good, as innocent of evil as brimstone and treacle, castor oil, or Gregory's powder.

In fact, it is a perfectly safe domestic remedy. For that reason I have no hesitation in commending it to the notice of the public in general, civil as well as military. In my opinion, if the use of it were universal throughout the army at the front there

GUNPOWDER AS A WAR REMEDY

would be infinitely fewer septic wounds among our wounded, and those wounds which become septic would heal in a vastly shorter space of time.

It may be asked how I can be so certain, seeing that I hold no official position in the Army or Navy, and have no opportunity of putting the remedy personally to the test of practice on a large scale. In reply, let me say that in medicine, as in warfare, the chance of success very often lies in an intelligent anticipation of the enemy's intentions and capabilities.

An ounce of wisdom is often worth many tons of experience. When cholera invaded Europe a little over a century ago the medical world was divided into two camps; the followers of Hahnemann on the one side, and all the rest on the other. Before the epidemic arrived reports of cases of the disease were bought and published.

From the symptoms described Hahnemann was able to name the remedies that were likely to be called for.

Consequently, his party, who exercised intelligent anticipation of what was to come, were all ready for action when the invasion occurred.

The other party, who may be called the party of the "Wait-and-Sees," never were ready, and lost over 70 percent of their patients, whilst the homoeopaths saved over 70 percent of theirs. In our Services, so far as I know, there are only Surgeon-captains, Surgeon-majors, Surgeon-colonels, and Surgeon-generals.

GUNPOWDER AS A WAR REMEDY

If there is such a person as a Physician-general I must confess I never heard of him.

But whilst surgery is paramount in war practice, and has reached a very high pitch of perfection, physicians' work is very necessary also, and I believe this branch of practice is not by any means so fully developed as he branch that belongs to mechanical surgery.

It is for this reason that I offer this contribution to the neglected branch, and I do not think any surgeon could object to such of his patients as might like to do so treating themselves to a few tablets of Gunpowder 3X.

THE END

www.ingramcontent.com/pod-product-compliance
Lightning Source LLC
Chambersburg PA
CBHW061454180526
45170CB00004B/1706